50 natural ways to
stay young

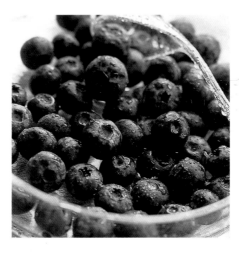

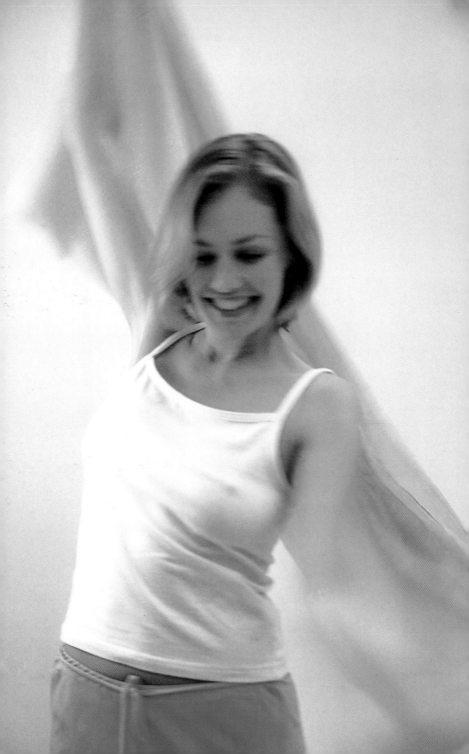

50 natural ways to
stay young

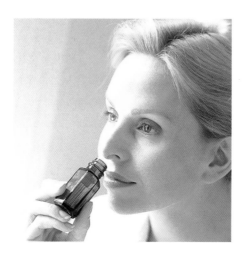

Tracey Kelly

LORENZ BOOKS

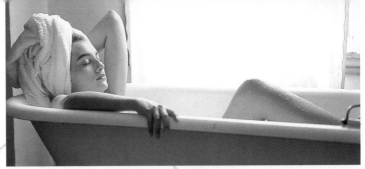

contents

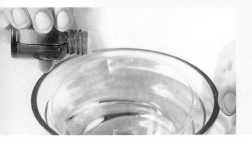

50 natural ways to...

stay young

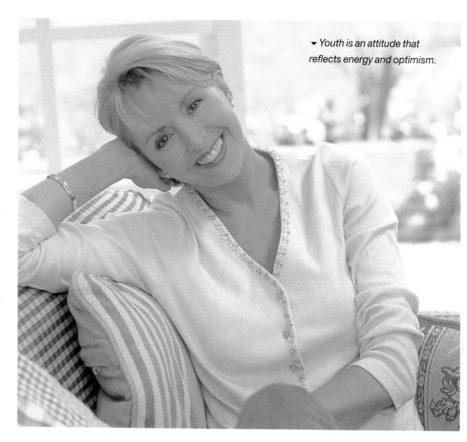

▼ Youth is an attitude that reflects energy and optimism.

introduction

As the population of the developed world enjoys an ever-increasing life span, more and more people are starting to reassess their approach to living and growing older. But growing older doesn't have to follow the traditional definition of aging – "aging" is what happens when we adopt destructive health habits and pessimistic mind sets.

It is possible to enjoy being forty, fifty or eighty years old and still be youthful; it all comes down to your attitude – and how well you take care of yourself. There are ways of staying younger than your chronological age, and many people achieve this by watching what they eat and how they exercise, sleep, relate to other people and deal with life's challenges. When you stop and consider that the wisdom you have gleaned from experience can benefit others, it makes sense to care for yourself, body and soul, to make the most of what you can offer the world.

water power

Probably the most essential ingredient for running the body's systems at optimal levels is water. Playing a major part in digesting foods and absorbing nutrients, water must be replenished almost constantly for the body to stay young and healthy – it is the one thing we cannot live without for very long.

The average person living in a temperate climate needs around eight large glasses of water a day – more in hotter climates or when exercising. Tea and coffee do not count in this quota. Drinking this amount will not only help keep your weight down, it will flush toxins out of the system, leaving your skin glowing – and beautiful skin is the most obvious indicator of youth and vigour.

food and exercise

Research into longevity has shown that by slowly reducing calories consumed over a period of years, the human life span can be prolonged. A diet high in fruit, vegetables and fibre and low in saturated fats is also beneficial. This doesn't mean that you can never enjoy high-calorie treats – only that it is best to modify your eating habits and keep an eye on sound nutrition most of the time.

Exercise works not only to boost the metabolism, so that the body responds from a younger fitness level, it also lifts the spirits, helping to energize and enthuse the mind, and keep depression at bay.

▾ *Replace your tea and coffee intake with refreshing herbal teas.*

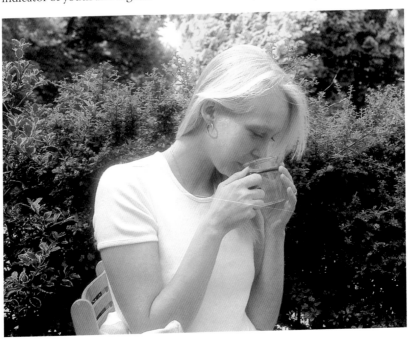

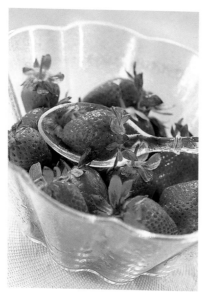

term heavy smoker. Their skin is sallow, teeth and lips yellow, and they may cough and get short of breath running up stairs. Kicking the habit is the best way to prevent lung disease.

supplemental help

As more research into aging is carried out, new information on beneficial substances comes to light. Many can be manufactured by the body, but the modern diet does not provide the necessary nutrients. Also, larger quantities of substances such as glucosamine sulphate – derived from seashells, which we do not normally eat – can be beneficial, in this case, protecting joints and cartilage. The antioxidant effects of tea polyphenols, grapeseed extract and co-enzyme Q-10 can work rejuvenating wonders.

soul food

Knowing when to ask for help is an important part of living in a society. No one is perfect or omnipotent, and sharing your problems – and joys – with family, friends and partners is helpful both for you and for them; giving is as important as receiving. Likewise, developing a sense of your own identity – exploring your feelings, thoughts and creativity – is crucial for wellbeing. Seeing yourself as a spiritual entity in the grand scheme of things puts your place in the world into perspective, and provides a good vantage point for a long and happy life.

changing habits

There is no doubt that avoiding eating certain foods, moderating your alcohol intake and giving up smoking are just as important as good nutrition and proper sleep. Reducing your fat and sugar intake is essential, as excesses overload the system, leading to imbalances and diseases such as diabetes and heart conditions. It is a good idea to cut out processed foods too – heating destroys crucial enzymes, and chemicals are often added.

Alcohol can play havoc with the system, especially as you grow older – drinking places stress on the liver, impairs the uptake of nutrients and damages cells. Cigarette smoking is one of the most destructive things you can do to your body, and one of the quickest ways to accelerate aging. You may think that it helps you to stay thin, or increases enjoyment of social activity – but take one look at a long-

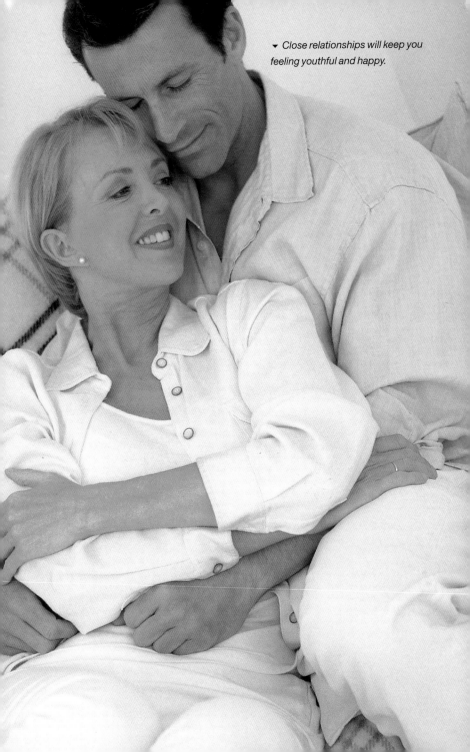

▾ *Close relationships will keep you feeling youthful and happy.*

anti-aging
treatments

This book outlines fundamental ways in which you can help stay the aging process. Sections on low-calorie and raw-fruit diets describe the foundations of nutritious eating, and information on choosing proteins, healthy fats, fibre and minerals completes the overall picture.

Supplements – from important antioxidants to brain-boosting herbs such as gingko biloba – can give your health and appearance a real boost. Calcium helps stave off osteoporosis, and B vitamins rejuvenate both mind and body.

Exercise is just as important as diet: included is information on aerobics and anaerobics, yoga and Tai Chi. Learning to deal effectively with stress and depression is a key to longevity, as are positive thinking, getting enough sleep and treating yourself to rejuvenating therapies.

Finally, enjoy the company of other people, have fun and develop a strong sense of your own identity and spirituality to be sure of the lengthiest and most fulfilled of lives.

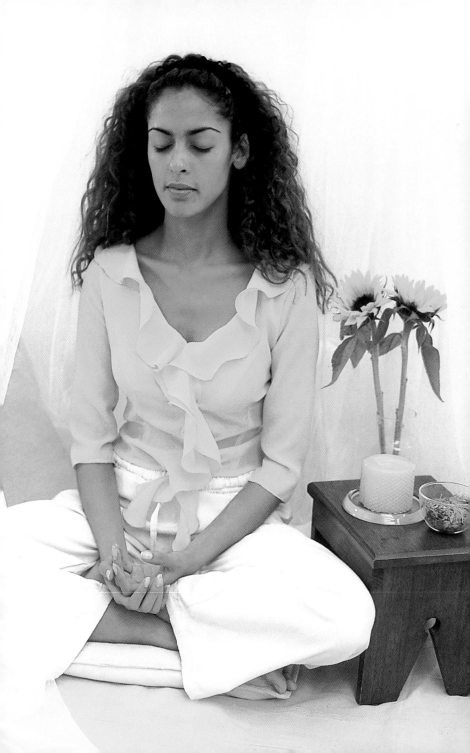

1 low-calorie diet

Research into longevity has shown that by reducing the total number of calories consumed daily, you can effectively prolong life – retaining health and youthful looks in the process.

Overeating is one of the worst age accelerators – it places stress on all of the body's systems, as digestion burns up extra energy that could be used for other functions. In addition, excess food causes weight gain, and excess fat is implicated in many age-onset diseases, such as heart disease and diabetes. This all boils down to one simple conclusion: if you eat less, you will live longer.

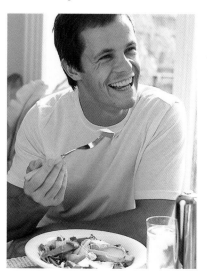

▲ Swapping high-calorie foods for more raw foods such as salads may extend your life.

important biomarkers

Biomarkers are factors that indicate how much younger you are physiologically than your chronological age. They include skin dryness, greying hair and blood cholesterol. Research with laboratory animals found great improvements when the animals were put on reduced-calorie diets; they lived longer, healthier lives than those who ate what they wanted.

slow decrease

Eating less does not mean skimping on nutrition – it means replacing high-calorie foods containing excess fats and sugars with raw, nutritious foods. It is suggested that, starting in middle age, the anti-aging diet should involve decreasing the amount of calories consumed to 60% of what you would normally eat – gradually, over a period of five to seven years.

This means reducing calories to 1,800 for men and 1,300 for women; slightly more for very active people. This controlled undernutrition effectively lowers body temperature and decreases metabolic rate, two major factors in increased longevity.

2 raw power

Following a diet high in raw foods – particularly fruit – is an achievable way to help you stay young. The enzymes in fresh, "live" foods act to keep the body's systems working at premium levels.

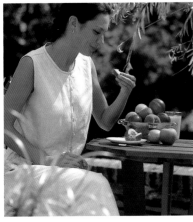

▲ *Eat fresh fruits slowly, chewing many times to release beneficial enzymes.*

When food is cooked, important enzymes are destroyed, so eating it raw, or juicing it for drinking immediately, ensures optimum levels of nutrients. Evidence suggests that a diet made up of 50% raw fruit can lengthen the life span. In fact, age researchers claim that a diet with 70% raw fruit and vegetables may actually begin to reverse the aging process: the body becomes leaner; wrinkles appear smoother and all-important brain function improves considerably.

TOP FRUITS

Although all fruits are good, some are particularly potent anti-agers. Choose organic fruits where possible, as they are free from pesticides – and they taste better.

• **Apples** Excellent detoxifiers with antiseptic qualities, which strengthen the immune system. Apples also contain pectin, which binds heavy metals such as lead and mercury and carries them out of the body.

• **Kiwi fruit** Containing double the vitamin C of oranges, twice as much vitamin E as an avocado, and a rich store of potassium, kiwis are wonderful.

• **Berries** Blackberries, blueberries, blackcurrants and black grapes contain phytochemicals known as flavonoids, potent antioxidants that protect against damage caused by free radicals.

• **Lemons** Very effective at flushing toxins from the system.

• **Dates and figs** Rich in calcium, iron and potassium, these are also good for digestion.

3 vital vegetables

Providing minerals, bioflavonoids, antioxidants, phytochemicals and protein, vegetables are essential for rejuvenating cell growth – and they make a delicious, colourful feast.

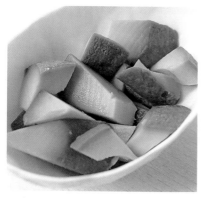

▲ *Avocado is an excellent source of skin-enhancing vitamin E and unsaturated fat.*

youth givers

Carrots are possibly the most beneficial of anti-aging vegetables. As well as cleansing, nourishing and stimulating the whole body, their rich supply of betacarotene has been found to lower the risk of cancer – eating just one medium-sized carrot per day can halve the risk of lung cancer. Other orange vegetables such as pumpkin, squash and sweet potatoes are also high in betacarotene.

Avocados are a good source of monounsaturated fat, which may help the body to reduce levels of "bad" cholesterol. A good source of vitamin E, avocado can help prevent skin aging, and its rich potassium content staves off fluid retention and high blood pressure.

green vegetation

Broccoli, cauliflower, Brussels sprouts, cabbage and watercress supply a toxin- and cancer-fighting cocktail of phytochemicals, and stimulate the liver. Broccoli has a plentiful supply of many B and C vitamins, and minerals such as calcium, folate, iron, potassium and zinc, and spinach contains a vast amount of minerals and antioxidants.

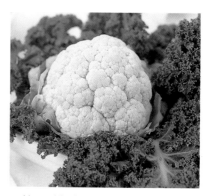

▲ *Vegetables in the* Brassica *family, such as cauliflower, help to prevent cancer.*

4 health-giving fish

Choosing from a variety of fish provides you with vital protein, minerals, vitamins and Omega 3 fatty acids. White fish is low in fat, while oily fishes such as tuna and mackerel are rich in vitamins A and D.

This tasty mackerel recipe is rich in Omega 3 fatty acids, which help prevent coronary heart disease and leave the skin clear and glowing.

moroccan spiced mackerel
serves 4
150ml/^{1}/$_4$ pint sunflower oil
15ml/1 tbsp paprika
5–10ml/1–2 tsp chilli powder
10ml/2 tsp ground cumin
10ml/2 tsp ground coriander
2 garlic cloves, crushed
juice of 2 lemons
salt and freshly ground black pepper
30ml/2 tbsp chopped mint leaves
30ml/2 tbsp chopped
    coriander (cilantro) leaves
4 fresh mackerel, cleaned
mint sprigs, to garnish

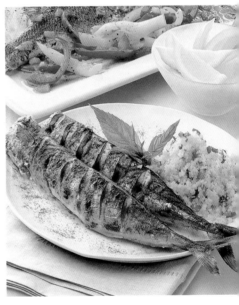

Whisk together the oil, spices, garlic and lemon juice. Season, then stir in the chopped mint and coriander to make a spicy marinade. Use a sharp knife to make a few diagonal slashes on either side of each mackerel.

Pour the marinade into a shallow non-metallic dish. Place the mackerel in the dish and spoon the marinade into the slashes, so that they absorb as much as possible. Cover the dish and leave to marinate for 3 hours. Preheat the grill to medium–high heat.

Transfer the fish to a rack set over a grilling pan and grill for 5–7 minutes, turning the fish once and basting several times. Serve the mackerel hot or cold, garnished with mint sprigs. Herb couscous or brown rice make good anti-aging accompaniments.

5 powerful proteins

Protein is essential for life, but only a very small amount is needed each day. Too much can contribute to a variety of health problems as you get older, including osteoporosis.

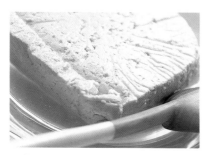

▲ Soya products such as tofu can be cooked as nutritious meat substitutes.

Most of us eat more protein that we need – estimates for requirements vary, but the range is from 5–10% of our total calorie intake. For best anti-aging results, try replacing at least some of your animal proteins with lower-fat plant proteins.

meat and poultry

Although red meat is a source of readily absorbed iron, zinc and B vitamins, it contains toxins, drugs and pesticides and is high in saturated fat. Eat only in moderation and choose lean cuts to reduce harmful fat intake. A good source of quality protein, B vitamins and iron, poultry is low in fat if the skin is removed, but should still be eaten sparingly. Choose organic, free-range poultry to ensure it is healthy, nutritious and cruelty-free.

dairy products

Yogurt is the most beneficial dairy product as it is non-mucus-forming and contains *Lactobacillus acidophilus*, which increases beneficial bacteria in the intestines and neutralizes excess hydrochloric acid in the stomach. Whole milk and cheese are mucus-forming (causing nasal congestion) and high in saturated fat, but may be consumed in moderation.

pulses

Beans and legumes such as lentils, pinto and mung beans, chick peas and soya beans are excellent sources of plant protein. Use dry beans in cooking, as processing, in all but a few exceptions, adds sugar and salt – they can be used to make delicious stews, soups and casseroles.

Tofu has been used in Chinese and Japanese cuisine for centuries – and the resulting reduction in saturated fats has been implicated in the lower incidence of cancers in these cultures.

6 fibre-rich grains

Providing fibre, carbohydrates, protein and minerals, grains have been a major part of the human diet for thousands of years. When eaten in whole form, they are potent anti-agers.

Eaten in moderation, grains are said to promote age reversal due to their rich supply of vitamins B and E, EFAs and lecithin, which helps to oxygenate the tissues. By absorbing impurities in the blood, fibre reduces levels of low-density lipoprotein and cholesterol levels, important in the prevention of heart disease.

Choose from a selection of unprocessed whole grains, including brown rice, oats, barley, millet, rye, buckwheat and quinoa. Containing soluble and insoluble fibre, grains are fundamental in the prevention of constipation, colon and rectal cancers. Research has shown that they also help prevent heart disease.

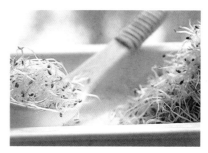

▲ Alfalfa sprouts are delicious and nutritious added to salads and sandwiches.

oat sense

An important anti-ager and easy to digest, a bowl of hot oats quickly helps cholesterol exit the body, and leaves the complexion glowing. Oats also act as a tonic for the nervous system, and stabilize sugar metabolism.

super sprouts

Sprouted grains contain many times the nutrient levels of unsprouted grains. They are the richest source of vitamins, minerals and enzymes – sprouted oats contain 1,000 times as much vitamin B as unsprouted.

Buy sprouts from health food stores, or it is easy to make your own from alfalfa, mung and other beans.

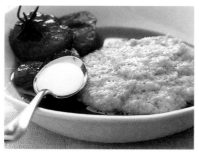

▲ Start the day with oat porridge and fruit for a supply of slow-burning energy.

7 antioxidant juices

Juicing fresh fruits provides you with antioxidant enzymes that serve to protect your cells from damaging free radicals. For maximum benefit, drink the juice directly after preparing.

By drinking fresh juice, you will retain all the important youth-enhancing, antioxidant enzymes contained in the fruit. Excellent for kick-starting the digestive system, the following high-energy drink is delicious at breakfast. You may also wish to create your own blends from combinations of papaya, mango, cantaloupe melon and white, green or black grapes – all are very beneficial.

pink vitality
serves 1
1 peach or nectarine
225g/8oz strawberries
30ml/2tbsp lemon juice

Cut the peach or nectarine into quarters around the stone (pit) and pull the fruit apart. Cut the flesh into rough chunks, then hull the strawberries. Juice all the fruit using a juicer, or blend in a blender for a thick juice with pulp. Stir in the lemon juice and drink immediately.

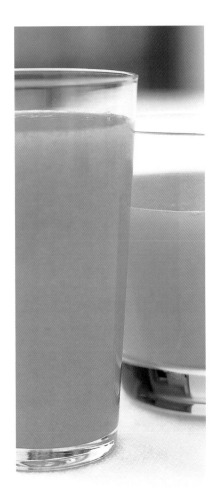

▸ *A blend of peach, strawberries and lemon juice makes a delicious drink rich in antioxidants.*

For a rejuvenating, caffeine-free, beverage, steep a teaspoon of chamomile, peppermint, fennel or mixed spices in boiling water for five minutes. Strain and enjoy.

9 essential fats

Contrary to popular belief, it is important to eat a variety of fats daily. If you learn the difference between "good" and "bad" fats, your body will reap the benefits – now and in the future.

Choosing the right fat is important for sustaining vitality as the body ages. Plant oils provide essential fatty acids (EFAs) and vitamin E, beneficial for heart and skin. High in unsaturated fats, olive, sunflower and grapeseed oils are all good choices. Often called the "king of oils", olive oil's tried and tested benefits in the Mediterranean diet include protection against heart disease. Some essential substances are lost from oils that are heated during processing, so look for organic, extra virgin olive oil and cold-pressed oils.

fats to avoid

Saturated fats – butter, cream, meat fats, palm and coconut oils – should be eaten in moderation, as they can raise cholesterol levels and clog the arteries. Processed foods such as "fast foods", cakes and biscuits often use hydrogenated fats, which are also saturated and are linked with cancer.

Omega magic

Foods and supplements with essential fatty acids (EFAs) can make dramatic improvements to skin tone and joint flexibility. Supplements with fish or flax oils contain Omegas 3, 6 and 9, which help the skin produce new elastin and collagen, making it firmer and more youthful. High in gamma-linoleic acid (GLA), evening primrose oil helps to regulate the hormones and control rheumatoid arthritis.

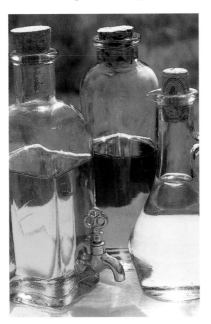

◄ Cold-pressed oils, such as olive and sunflower, are best for the anti-aging dieter.

10 mineral-packed nuts & seeds

Nuts and seeds contain compact energy in the form of protein, fats, carbohydrates and myriad minerals. To reap their excellent, youth-preserving benefits, include several types in your daily diet.

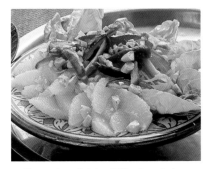

▲ *For a mineral-rich addition to salads, throw in a handful of your favourite nuts.*

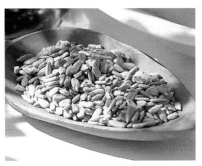

▲ *Sunflower seeds are delicious and easy to carry for a quick afternoon pick-me-up.*

go nuts

Most varieties of nuts are good sources of minerals, especially walnuts and brazil nuts. Although high in calories, walnuts are rich in iron, zinc, potassium, magnesium, copper and selenium. Almonds, peanuts, cashews, hazelnuts and pine nuts also offer excellent health benefits.

Adding nuts to your diet in small quantities can work to enhance the effectiveness of your digestive and immune systems and improve the quality of your skin and hair. Though high in fat, they actually help reduce cholesterol levels because the fat they contain is polyunsaturated.

Nuts stay fresh longer when bought in the shell and used as needed. They can be eaten on their own, or added to porridge, breads, casseroles and salads. Never eat rancid nuts – they have been linked to cancer-causing free radicals.

grab a seed snack

Seeds such as pumpkin, sunflower and sesame offer high nutritional values with slightly fewer calories than nuts. Sunflower seeds, for example, are a good source of vitamin B3 (niacin), known to fight depression, high blood pressure, circulatory problems and asthma. Add to breads and salads.

11

sulphur-rich eggs & garlic

An important protector against radiation and chemical pollutants, sulphur has also been shown to prolong the life span of animals. Eggs and garlic are both excellent sources.

amino acid protection

Sulphur-based amino acids such as methionine, cysteine and taurine are important antioxidant nutrients – they scavenge free radicals, neutralize toxic waste and help process proteins. They also help to protect against the effects of radiation from X-rays, mobile phones, power lines and low-level nuclear radiation, to which we are increasingly exposed.

food sources

As well as containing the most complete nutrition of any food – including protein, iron, zinc and

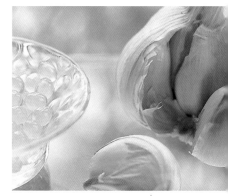

▲ Garlic may be taken in its natural form (cloves) or as a deodorized supplement.

▼ Fresh, free-range eggs are an excellent source of sulphur and many other nutrients.

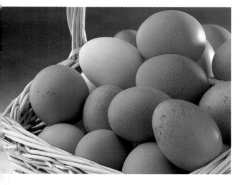

vitamins A, E and B complex – eggs are a rich source of sulphur, with 65mg each. The human body contains around 140g of sulphur and almost a gram is lost every day.

Garlic – like other members of the *Allium* family, such as onions – also contains a high level of sulphur. In addition, eating a clove of garlic a day (which may be raw or cooked) helps protect against heart disease – it reduces cholesterol levels and assists blood-thinning more effectively than aspirin, thus reducing the risk of heart attack and stroke.

12 cell-boosting vitamin C

Vitamin C is one of the most important nutrients in cell repair and therefore a potent anti-aging agent. Together with vitamin E and betacarotene, it is one of the "big three" antioxidants.

An essential nutrient for maintaining a resilient immune system, vitamin C assists with tissue growth, the healing of wounds, and the prevention of blood clotting and bruising. It is a powerful antioxidant which, when taken with betacarotene and vitamin E, helps curtail the effects of pollution. It reduces facial wrinkles and promotes a smooth complexion, due to its role in maintaining collagen, which binds cells together.

high–C foods and supplements
Vitamin C is ideally sourced from the food you eat, and many fruits and vegetables are high in it. Choose from a variety of berries, citrus fruits, kiwi fruits, green leafy vegetables, guavas, tomatoes, apples, melons and peppers to include in your daily diet.

When choosing supplements, try to find a brand with bioflavonoids, which work in conjunction with vitamin C. As it is not retained by the body, time–released vitamin C offers most benefit, allowing slow leaching into the digestive tract. Many health advisers recommend 200–500mg a day to keep infections at bay.

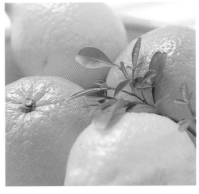

▲ *Citrus fruits such as oranges are an important source of vitamin C.*

▼ *Versatile tomatoes contain a good supply of vitamin C and other antioxidants.*

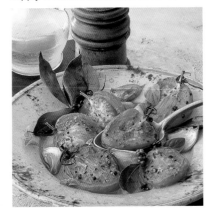

13 health-preserving vitamin E

Vitamin E is an essential fat-soluble substance containing several antioxidant compounds that help the body to fight free radicals and boost immunity to aid in the prevention of disease.

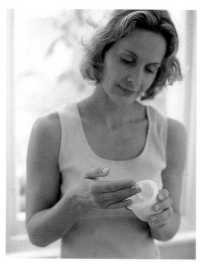

▲ *Vitamin E creams and oils help to heal burns and soothe dry, damaged skin.*

In laboratory tests, vitamin E has been shown to slow the aging process and enhance immune functions. Those with higher levels of this important antioxidant get fewer infections than people with average levels. Vitamin E is also known to help prevent degenerative diseases such as heart disease, arthritis, diabetes and cancer. It keeps your skin looking younger and glowing, and helps keep wrinkles

at bay. Vitamin E deficiency is rare, but signs include thread veins and slow-healing wounds.

sources of vitamin E
Vitamin E is found in many foods: nuts, sunflower and pumpkin seeds, cold-pressed oils, vegetables, spinach, grains, asparagus, avocado, beef,

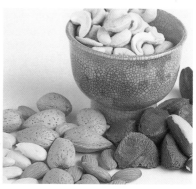

▲ *Nuts such as almonds and cashews are a good source of healing vitamin E.*

seafood, apples, carrots and celery. As a supplement, vitamin E is best taken with betacarotene, vitamin C and selenium. Experts recommend no more than 600–1,200IU daily. Always build up to higher doses slowly.

14 protective betacarotene

An important antioxidant in preventing age degeneration of the cells and tissues, betacarotene appears to fight several forms of cancer as well as offering many other benefits.

Betacarotene – or pro-vitamin A – is converted to vitamin A by the body from foods, but unlike vitamin A, it is not toxic in high doses. A plant substance, this antioxidant boosts the immune system and has been shown to slow many types of cancer.

In studies, it was shown that women who had eaten betacarotene-rich foods for 18 months had a lower

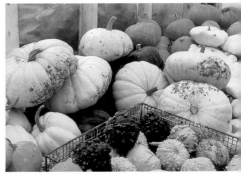

▲ *Pumpkins and the many varieties of squash are rich sources of betacarotene.*

risk of cancer – but those who benefited most had been eating these foods for 20 years or more.

beta benefits
Betacarotene promotes growth and strong bones; it strengthens teeth, hair, skin and gums and helps the respiratory systems resist infections. It also helps prevent night blindness and improves weak eyesight.

It is found in many fruits and vegetables, including carrots, pumpkins, squashes, spinach, broccoli, cantaloupe, sweet potatoes, apricots, peaches, Brussels sprouts and oranges.

▼ *Carrots have been found to reduce the risk of breast cancer after the menopause.*

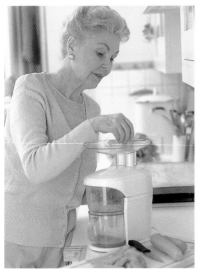

15 essential B & K vitamins

Because of their role in releasing energy from food, providing the body with steady nutrients, B group and K vitamins are vital. Eat a range of vitamin B-rich foods, as they work in tandem with each other.

the B group

When adopting a balanced anti-aging diet, consuming a variety of foods that contain all of the B vitamins is important. B group vitamins are found in large quantities in liver and yeast, and they exist singly or in combinations in all of the food groups. Eat seeds, nuts, legumes, dairy products, meats, fish and eggs.

Vitamins B6, B12 and folate are important in staving off the effects of aging, because they affect methylation, an essential chemical process that helps maintain the body's DNA and protein. They are also believed to

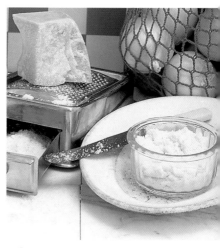

▲ Dairy products contain many B group vitamins; yogurt is also rich in vitamin K.

protect the heart and brain from age-related damage, balance the hormones and prevent depression.

the K concept

Vitamin K has excellent anti-aging properties. It is believed to reduce the risk of osteoporosis, improve bone health, strengthen gums and reduce the risk of heart disease. Sources include broccoli, Brussels sprouts, liver, yogurt, beans, soya and lean red meat.

▼ Nuts, legumes and seeds such as pumpkin all contain B complex vitamins.

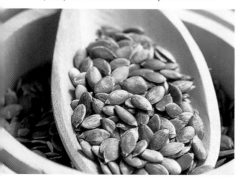

16 bone-protecting calcium

Important for strong bones and teeth, adequate amounts of calcium and vitamin D help prevent the onset of osteoporosis, one of the most significant age-related illnesses, especially in women.

calcium count

Eating a diet that is rich in calcium is invaluable in protecting the body from osteoporosis – a disease in which the bones become fragile and brittle. It is important to start as young as possible – fortifying the body with plenty of calcium in the teenage years and young adulthood can reduce the risk of developing the disease in later years.

Foods that contain rich supplies of calcium include almonds, sesame seeds, beans, tofu and dairy products such as milk, cheese and yogurt. Other foods that offer good supplies include fish such as sprats, whitebait and sardines, particularly when their bones are eaten as well as the flesh.

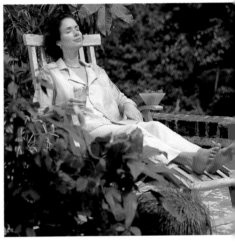

▲ *Spending time in the sunlight will ensure that your body receives enough vitamin D.*

THE SUNLIGHT VITAMIN

Vitamin D is also crucial for strong bones, and some exposure to sunlight is essential for boosting body supplies. Extra vitamin D can be obtained from sea fish such as salmon, sardines and herring, from fish liver oils and egg yolks, or by taking it in tablet form.

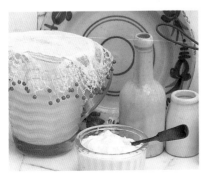

◀ *Dairy products such as milk, yogurt and cheese are good sources of calcium.*

17 super antioxidants

Grapeseed extract and tea polyphenols are antioxidants with strong life-preserving qualities. You can get your supply by eating grapes and drinking tea, or by taking supplements.

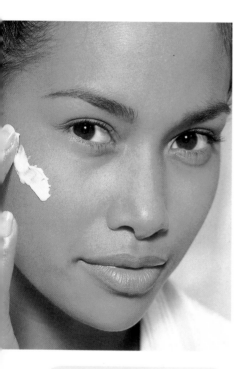

grapeseed extract

A bioflavonoid that acts to keep capillaries and connective tissue in good condition, grapeseed extract is a potent free radical scavenger. It is very beneficial for smokers, those exposed to second-hand smoke and exercisers, all of whom are bombarded by free radicals (exercisers are at risk due to their faster metabolisms). You can chew on the seeds of white or green grapes, or take supplements.

tea polyphenols

Due to its high polyphenol content, green tea is a goldmine of cancer-fighting properties. Polyphenols seem to deter cancer in three ways: they stop the cancer cells from forming, increase the body's detoxification defenses, and prevent cancer cells from growing. They also act as skin detoxifiers and skin-aging inhibitors.

Black tea contains about half the polyphenol content of green tea, but is still useful drunk in small quantities. White tea, which is dried in sunlight and is very expensive, has the highest level of polyphenols of all the teas – about three times that of green tea.

COSMETIC MAGIC
In addition to ingesting these antioxidants, using them externally also helps protect the skin from damage. Many commercial skin ranges use tea polyphenols and grapeseed extract in their moisturizers and cosmetics.

18 herbal brain boosters

Ginkgo biloba and vinpocetine are natural plant substances that are used therapeutically to boost brain power and delay the onset of age-related memory loss and other problems.

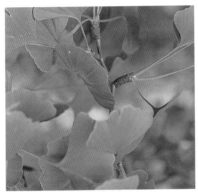

▲ *Memory-enhancing ginko biloba.*

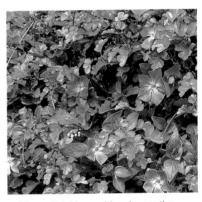

▲ *The periwinkle provides vinpocetine.*

ginkgo biloba

The earliest known medicinal use of ginkgo – often called "The Fountain of Youth" because the plant has survived 200 million years – dates back to 2800BC. Today it is one of the most popular herbal remedies in the world, due largely to its role in improving brain function. Ginkgo is used to combat memory loss, and to treat the early stages of Alzheimer's disease and depression in the elderly. This amazing plant also aids poor circulation, erectile problems and hearing loss, and it is used as a long-term therapy for stroke victims.

vinpocetine

Derived from the periwinkle plant, the action of vinpocetine is similar to that of gingko biloba. It works to improve mental function by increasing the blood circulation to the brain, thus improving the way the brain uses glucose and oxygen. It also enhances the function of neurotransmitters such as serotonin, which regulates emotions, mood, sleep and appetite. (Serotonin levels often fall when people are under stress.) Vinpocetine guards against ear problems such as tinnitus (ringing in the ears) and vertigo (dizziness).

19 age-defying supplements

Certain substances occur naturally in the body, but either exist in small quantities or their production declines from an early age. Supplements can provide dramatic anti-aging effects.

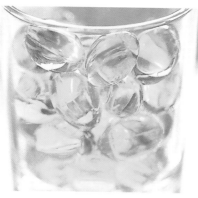

▲ *Supplements are a good way to boost levels of co-enzyme Q-10 and carnosine.*

co-enzyme Q-10

This super-nutrient, also called ubiquinone, is an antioxidant with a huge number of anti-aging benefits. Its most important effects include lowering blood pressure, boosting the immune system, protecting the brain and eyes from damage, and helping to prevent heart disease.

Co-enzyme Q-10 fights aging at the mitochondrial level in the cells, and may dramatically reverse the effects of aging and a poor diet. Although it is a natural substance made by the body, the production of co-enzyme Q-10 declines around the age of 20, and many people take it as a supplement. Food sources include trout, sardines, mackerel, nuts and soya.

carnosine

An antioxidant amino acid found in brain, muscle and eye tissue, carnosine stabilizes and protects cell membranes, and scavenges free radicals from both external pollutants and internal chemical reactions. It helps fight the process of glycosylation – a dangerous coupling of sugar molecules to body protein – which causes widespread damage and aging. Food sources include lean red meat and chicken.

▼ *Co-enzyme Q-10 is present in small amounts in mackerel and other oily fish.*

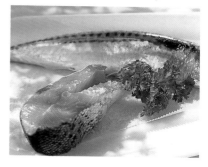

By eating just three or four **brazil nuts** a day, you will get your quota of **selenium**, which helps to prevent cancer and may **extend** life.

21 yoga for flexibility

Anti-aging experts agree that yoga is the top exercise for promoting longevity. It fosters balance, control and peace of mind, and lends the body great suppleness and fluidity.

Yoga works to build up a store of physical health, while keeping the body and mind cleansed and fit. The asanas (exercises) help in the removal of toxins, circulation of the blood and the smooth function of the organs.

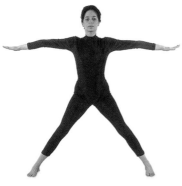

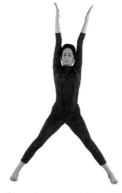

1 To perform the Warrior, stand with your feet together and arms at your side. Inhale deeply and jump the feet 120cm/4ft apart. Extend the arms.

2 Turn the palms up and stretch your arms over your head. Keep the arms parallel, elbows tight and palms facing each other.

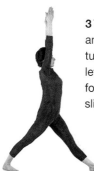

3 Turn right leg 45° in, and left foot 90° out, turning hips to the left. Bring right hip forwards and left hip slightly back.

4 Exhale; bend left leg into a right angle, stretching whole body. Take head back and stretch for 20–30 seconds. Repeat.

22 heart-enhancing aerobics

The benefits of aerobic exercise are many, but the most important for anti-aging is its very positive effect on the heart and cardiovascular system, keeping the body fit and "tuned".

Any exercise that increases the respiratory rate and boosts the heart rate from 60–80% of its capacity is called aerobic, meaning "sustained by oxygen". Tennis, jogging, cycling, dancing and swimming are all excellent aerobic sports. Perhaps the easiest and most accessible is walking: it can be done anywhere, needs no special equipment and varies endlessly with different locations and terrains. Aerobics classes with planned routines are available at most night schools and gyms, and some target specific age groups and fitness levels.

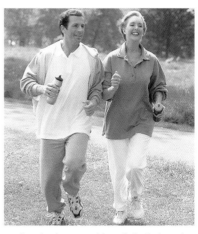

▲ Jogging is an aerobic activity that can be enjoyed in the fresh air with a friend.

powerful advantages

Aerobic exercise burns fat, boosts the immune system and helps prevent the build-up of fatty deposits in the arteries. It enhances joint and muscle flexibility, and aids stamina, digestion and sleep – if you suffer at all from insomnia, this is your first port of call for a remedy. The body was designed for movement, and if it doesn't move, all of its systems suffer. The mind suffers too; exercise is a major ingredient in keeping mentally fit as well as physically active.

never too late

Recent studies have shown that even people who have not exercised for 20 years can benefit significantly from an aerobics regime. It is possible to gain the fitness levels of a younger body in a surprisingly short period of time, and the sooner you start, the sooner you will reap the rewards. Begin slowly, gradually building up your stamina, strength and suppleness. Consult your doctor if you are planning to start exercising after years of inactivity.

23 muscle-boosting anaerobics

Anaerobic exercise, where the muscles work at high intensity for short periods, is especially important because the body loses muscle tissue as it ages – up to about a third by the age of 65.

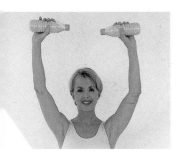

arm lifts
1 Stand with feet hip-width apart. Using weights if preferred, raise your arms above your head and circle round. Repeat 5 times. This lift is good for added flexibility and tone.

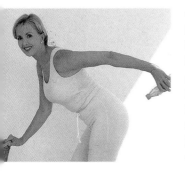

triceps curls
2 Place one hand on the back of a chair, then lean forwards. Holding a weight in the other hand, slowly lift it behind you in a smooth, controlled movement. Do 5 lifts, then repeat with the other arm.

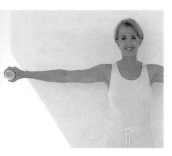

side lifts
3 Hold the weights at your sides, then slowly raise your arms to 90° to your body. Slowly lower your arms again, and repeat 5 times. This movement helps to tighten upper arms.

Working the muscles anaerobically improves muscle tone, posture and overall strength. This can be done through activities such as weight lifting, sprinting, squash and weight-bearing forms of yoga. Gyms have starter programmes for all ages and fitness levels, and personal trainers can help design a regime based around your own requirements.

arm workout
Keeping the arms well-toned, using light weights with many repetitions, will ease tension in the shoulders and neck and help prevent injuries such as RSI (Repetitive Strain Injury), a common problem for computer users, factory workers and musicians.

24 safe lifting

As you get older, innocent, everyday tasks can be a minefield of potential injuries. With a little care, movements such as bending, squatting, sitting, standing and lifting can be performed safely.

Back problems become increasingly common with age and inactivity, and many injuries are brought on by incorrect movement. This exercise will help you to re-train your body to support the lower back while bending and lifting loads. To avoid unnecessary strain on the back, stand as close to the load as possible and place your feet to either side of it.

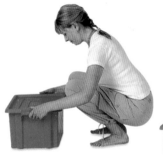

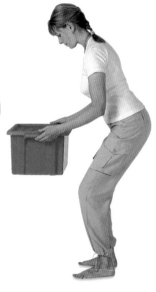

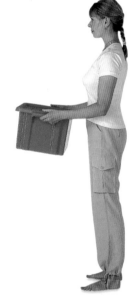

lifting a heavy object
1 To lift a heavy load safely, get as close to it as possible. Move into a squat by bending your knees and keeping your back straight and your feet firmly on the ground. Keep your head aligned with your back bone. Bend your arms so that your elbows are close to your body to help you lift.

2 Hold the load firmly without tensing the wrists. If the arms, wrists and hands are tense, you will lose the contact with your lower back.

3 Once you are holding the load as closely to your body as possible, slowly rise out of the squat and stand.

25 natural face lift

Tension held in the face can lead to wrinkles and sagging muscles as gravity comes into effect. By doing simple exercises each day, you can help retain the youthful elasticity of your features.

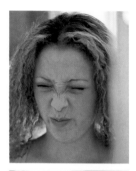

line eraser

1 Scrunch up your whole face for a few seconds, so that your nose is wrinkled, your forehead furrowed, and your eyes and mouth are tightly closed.

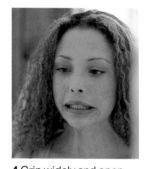

2 Now do the opposite: open your mouth and eyes as wide as you can (as if you are silently screaming) to release the tension in your throat and neck muscles.

4 Grin widely and open your eyes wide. Relax the eyes, hold and repeat the grin, this time tucking your chin in. Relax and repeat once more.

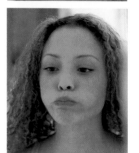

3 Relax your eyes for a moment. Close your mouth again, purse your lips and push your mouth up first to the left, and then to the right.

CHIN FIRMER
Using the backs of your hands alternately, pat the area beneath your chin using quick, stroking movements. Done for a few minutes every day, this will help to firm up slack skin and reduce signs of a double chin.

26 abdomen strengthener

The girdle of muscles in the abdomen supports the spine and torso. To keep fit, healthy and free from back pain, it is important to keep this area toned and strong with simple exercises.

When doing these sit-ups, lift your head and shoulders as one unit, never separately – roll up from the top of your head. It may help to imagine that you are holding a peach between your chin and chest, and try to keep this gap constant throughout. Be sure to keep your facial muscles relaxed and loose.

sit-ups

1 Lying flat on the floor with your arms by your sides and your palms down, bend your knees and keep your feet flat on the floor, a short distance apart and in line with your hips. Be sure to keep your lower abdomen tight by keeping the muscles contracted throughout the exercise.

2 Lift your head and shoulders upwards, exhaling as you rise, and push your fingertips towards your knees, keeping your arms straight.

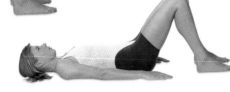

NOTE
With any exercise, is important to stop if you feel anything more than a mild sensation of muscle fatigue. Always work at your own pace and stop if you feel dizzy. Do not attempt to exercise when you are ill or feverish.

3 Lower your body back to the starting position, breathing in as you go down. When you get to the floor, do not allow yourself a chance to rest but repeat the movement from step 1.

27 balancing Tai Chi

An ancient martial art and active meditation, Tai Chi is practised daily by millions of Chinese – many very long-lived. It enhances balance and has a "grounding" effect on the nervous system.

The physical and mental aspects of Tai Chi are very closely entwined. In Chinese medicine and philosophy, the interdependence of mind, body and spirit is seen as crucial for one's well-being. In Tai Chi, the alertness, relaxed mind, softening and opening of the joints, balance and flow of chi (energy) evenly through the body are all equally important.

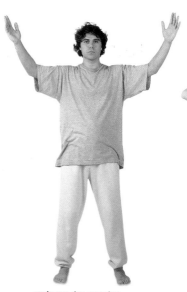

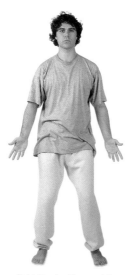

return to centre
1 As you breathe in, move your hands out to the sides in front of your body, and raise them slowly in a large circle, palms facing upwards.

2 As you exhale, lower your hands in front of the centre of your body, with your palms facing downwards.

3 At the bottom of the circle, turn your hands outwards again to begin a new circle with the new breath. Repeat several times until the movement is flowing.

28 deep breathing exercises

Proper breathing is important for a youthful system. It facilitates the movement of oxygen through the blood, "feeding" the cells, removing impurities and enhancing the body's energy flow.

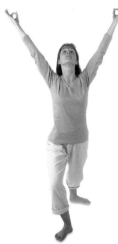

chest opening exercise

1 These exercises help to open up the chest to better facilitate deep breathing. Stand with your feet shoulder-width apart and your knees bent. Lift your arms out to the sides with your elbows bent, and make loose fists with your hands. Take a deep breath in, opening your chest by bringing your arms back as much as possible.

2 On exhaling, cross your arms in front of you, and relax your head down. Keeping your knees bent, press the area in between your shoulder blades backwards, and feel the muscles stretching. Empty your breath out completely. Repeat the exercise 4 or 5 times.

lung stretch
Link your index fingers and thumbs. Step forward with your right foot and reach up to the ceiling. Look up as you breathe in, and feel your chest expanding as your lungs fill with air.

Step back with your foot and relax your arms as you breathe out. Step forward again, this time with your left foot, and repeat the same movement. Repeat another 3 or 4 times.

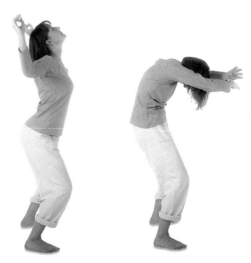

29 nourishing night cream

As the body matures, the skin becomes drier and loses elasticity. Moisturizing at night with a rich cream can help your face retain its youthful smoothness and rounded contours.

The delicate skin of the face is constantly exposed to the elements. To keep fine lines at bay, try this cosmetic, which uses a perfume-free base cream rich in vitamin E or evening primrose oil.

Jasmine and rose oils are added to help rehydrate the skin, while the frankincense oil helps to reduce wrinkles and restore tone to slack muscles. Good-quality essential oils can be obtained from health food stores, and there are many brands of prepared creams available.

▼ Use night cream only on cleansed skin or you will trap impurities, which can irritate.

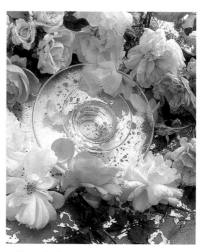

▲ Not only does rose essential oil help to rejuvenate the skin, its scent is heavenly.

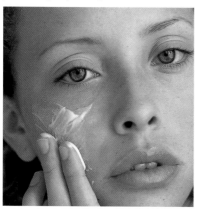

nourishing night cream
50g/2oz jar of unperfumed vitamin E
   or evening primrose oil cream
3 drops rose essential oil
2 drops frankincense essential oil
1 drop jasmine essential oil

Add the oils to the cream and mix with a clean metal spoon. After washing, apply small dabs to the forehead, cheeks, chin, nose and neck. Massage gently into the skin.

For a sensual treat, use 1 tablespoon almond oil plus 3 drops each rose and sandalwood oils, swirl into a warm bath and climb into a youthful indulgence.

31

gentle eye treatments

Tired, puffy eyes can occur for many reasons –
computer fatigue, lack of sleep or crying – making
you appear older. These home-made remedies will
refresh the delicate eye area and reduce swelling.

The following treatments involve lying down with your eyes closed for at least 15 minutes. This relaxation period is almost as important a part of the treatment as the compresses.

▾ Tea contains astringent tannin, making it ideal for a simple compress for tired eyes.

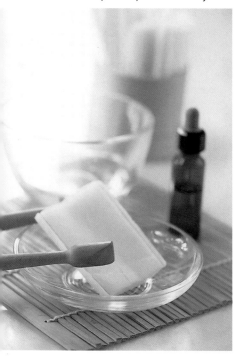

cooling cucumber
Place a cool slice of fresh organic cucumber over each eye and then relax. Cucumber works very gently to tone and refresh the skin around the eyes while reducing swelling.

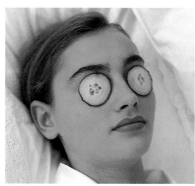

tea bag treatment
Ordinary tea contains tannin, which is astringent and tones the skin. Place a couple of Indian or African tea bags on a saucer and pour hot water over them. Cover with another saucer and refrigerate until cool. Gently squeeze the excess moisture from the bags, place them over your eyes, lie down and relax. Remove the tea bags and gently pat the skin dry before dabbing on a gentle moisturizer.

32 restorative hair mask

As hair ages, it tends to become drier and more brittle, especially grey hair that has been colour-treated. Applying a hair mask will help restore moisture and gloss to tired hair.

Deep conditioning of the hair will help promote shiny, lustrous locks. For a really rich, moisturizing treatment that adds body to dry or lank hair, try the following once every two or three weeks. As the ingredients are all natural, the preparation is safe to use even on tinted hair.

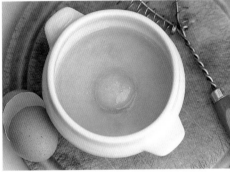

rich hair mask
1 egg yolk, lightly beaten
15ml/1 tbsp olive oil

Beat ingredients together. Work the mask into dry hair before washing and massage into the scalp. Gently comb or finger through, then wrap in a warm towel; leave for 20–30 minutes. Follow with a gentle shampoo, using a a final rinse of cool water.

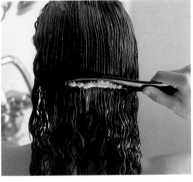

▲ *Use a wide-tooth comb to distribute the conditioner evenly through the strands.*

GREYING
At some stage during middle adulthood, the pigment formation in hair slows down and silver-grey strands begin to appear. The speed of the process is largely due to genetic factors, but foods containing vitamin B5 are said to help slow the onset of grey hair. Eating a wide selection of fruit, vegetables and nuts will ensure your hair is kept in optimum condition, whatever its colour.

33 skin sense

The youngest-looking people are those who eat fresh foods, drink plenty of water and shun the midday sun. Not only is this wise from a vanity point of view, it also helps prevent skin cancer.

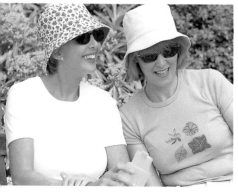

▲ Sun hats help prevent damage to skin.

As skin ages, it loses collagen and becomes drier, more "brittle" and thin, factors that lead to fine lines and wrinkles. The skin on the hands and face age faster due to exposure to the elements and pollutants, but there are ways that you can slow the process.

avoid UV light and smoke

The single most effective way to prevent premature skin aging is to protect your skin from the UV (ultraviolet) rays of the sun. Although a little sunshine is no bad thing, particularly as the body needs it to manufacture vitamin D, when out in bright sunlight, it is best to wear a hat and sunglasses, and use a sunscreen with an SPF (Sun Protection Factor) of at least 15, depending on your skin colour and type.

healthy tips

Water is important for healthy skin – it flushes out toxins and moisturizes from the inside. When skin is exposed to artificial heat in buildings, it can lose up to 2 litres/3 1/2 pints of water per day, so keep rehydrating. Eat fresh foods rich in vitamins A, C and E, betacarotene, selenium and zinc, and get good quality sleep each night.

FACIAL MOISTURIZING

There are a number of good facial creams and lotions available commercially, and constant advances in research mean that these often contain many of the latest known anti-aging ingredients, vitamins and antioxidants. Products containing alpha-hydroxy acids (AHAs) are said to combat some of the effects of aging by "sloughing off" the top layers of epidermis.

34 soothing hand cream

The hands are the most used part of the body – they tend to age faster due to exposure to water, detergent and the elements. This lotion will help heal and protect against chapped, dry skin.

Lavender contains over 200 active substances, and is perfect for use in moisturizers as it not only soothes and heals, but has a wonderful fragrance as well. By making your own hand cream, you ensure that the ingredients are fresh and free from chemical additives and preservatives. The materials needed for this recipe are available from most chemists.

▼ Lavender hand cream acts as a rejuvenating barrier that fights dryness caused by exposure to pollutants.

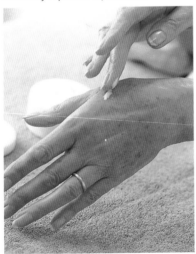

lavender moisturizer

20g/³/4oz cocoa butter
10ml/2tsp borax
175ml/6fl oz lavender water
75ml/5tbsp almond oil
20ml/4tsp beeswax granules
8 drops lavender essential oil
mixing bowl
saucepans
wooden spoon
glass jar

Measure out the cocoa butter, borax, lavender water, almond oil and beeswax granules in separate containers. Put the beeswax, cocoa butter and almond oil in a bowl set over a saucepan of simmering water. Stir well until the ingredients melt.

In a separate pan, dissolve the borax and lavender water by gently warming it. Add the lavender/borax mixture to the bowl; stir constantly. When the ingredients are thoroughly combined, take the mixture off the heat and allow it to cool. While still tepid, add the lavender oil and mix well. Pour the moisturizer into a glass jar and store in the refrigerator. Use within three weeks.

35 invigorating aromatherapy

Aromatherapy oils work by sending molecules to the brain's olfactory centre via the nostrils, or by being absorbed into the skin. They can have significant physiological and psychological effects.

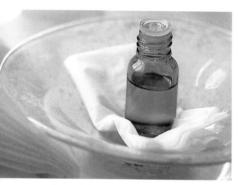

▲ Essential oils have many uses, from antidepressant to digestive stimulant.

anti-aging oils

Although there are no magic potions that will keep you young forever, certain plant essences can stimulate the growth of healthy new cells. The most effective are neroli and lavender.

Lavender is not only a powerful skin rejuvenator, it also helps balance both dry and greasy skins, and combats acne. Delicate neroli oil is used in many skincare products and is useful for dry and sensitive skin. It can also help the skin's elasticity, and improve the appearance of thread veins (common on older, thinner skin) and stretch marks.

oil dispersion

Essential oils can be used in a number of ways. Try placing a few drops in an oil burner to disperse throughout the room, or place on a tissue and sniff. You could also place a lightly impregnated piece of cloth or tissue inside your pillowcase at night.

Regular use of both lavender and neroli in baths and massage can help to maintain cellular reproduction at levels that naturally occur in younger people. Add a few drops of the oils to a very warm bath, or to a base oil such as almond for a relaxing massage. You can also experiment by adding the oils to face creams and body lotions.

OTHER USEFUL OILS
- **Rose** Antidepressant, sexual tonic, aphrodisiac.
- **Ylang ylang** Circulatory and respiratory stimulant, antispasmodic.
- **Black pepper** Analgesic, antidepressant, expectorant.
- **Ginger** Anticatarrhal, analgesic, digestive stimulant.
- **Myrrh** Anti-inflammatory, antiseptic, emotional sedative.

36 regenerative hydrotherapy

Water has been used as a healing aid throughout the centuries, in all cultures. By using hot or cold ablutions – or a combination – you can stimulate, cleanse and regenerate the body's systems.

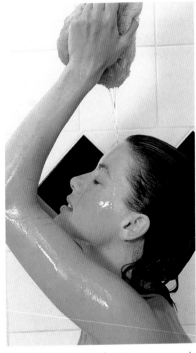

◀ *Cool, running water tightens and tones the skin and refreshes the whole body.*

vitality shower

Start by priming your body with a brief warm shower, until you feel the heat permeating your skin, but not so hot that you turn lobster red (very hot water damages skin tissue). Now turn on the cold tap, and direct the shower all over your body, from your face to your limbs, and down your torso and back, for 20–30 seconds.

Get out and pat yourself dry, then put on some warm clothes. If you cannot warm up afterwards, take another warm shower – do not risk giving yourself a chill.

anti-aging face affusion

Running water on the face stimulates the blood supply to the skin, leaving it more taut and fresh. Start by making sure your whole body is warm. Take the head off a shower attachment, and run cold water. Bending over the bath, rest your head on a rolled-up towel and let the stream of water flow gently over your face, in a circular motion, for three minutes. Pat dry.

As anyone who bathes in an open-air swimming pool knows, cold water is a wonderful tonic for the skin, leaving it glowing and healthy-looking. The positive stress of temperature change can make your immune system stronger and more resistant to illness, while giving you an energizing boost.

37 "spring clean" fast

Fasting is recommended by many anti-aging experts to cleanse the body, stimulate its systems and give the digestion a rest. This weekend fast is a gentle yet effective way to rejuvenate.

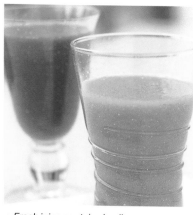

▲ *Fresh juice contains healing enzymes.*

People who fast periodically have been shown to have the tissues of a much younger body. Even after a short fast, improvements can be seen: facial lines soften, skin condition improves and eyes become brighter.

In this regime, plentiful fluids are combined with vegetables and fruits to rid the system of built-up impurities. Choose a weekend when you can allow yourself plenty of time for rest, relaxation and reflection. Book a massage and take some gentle exercise to stimulate the metabolism.

the fast
The evening before the fast, have a light, vegetable-based meal, such as soup or a green salad.

mornings
On rising, drink a cup of hot water with lemon juice to kick-start the liver. Prepare a fruit juice and dilute with water for breakfast. Eat a bunch of grapes or an apple mid-morning.

afternoons
Make up a fresh vegetable juice, such as carrot and spinach, and a large salad for lunch and drink plenty of mineral water. Do simple stretches all day.

evenings
Prepare a dinner of lightly steamed organic vegetables, sprinkled with fresh herbs and lemon juice, accompanied by brown rice. It is a good idea to end each day with relaxation techniques or meditation, followed by a warming bath.

Always consult a doctor or nutritionist if you plan a fast lasting longer than two days.

38 coping with depression

The likelihood of depression may increase as you get older, but there are ways to combat "feeling down". Recognizing the warning signs can help you take self-help action sooner.

Depression is different from the unhappy mood you may have when something goes wrong in your life. It is longer lasting and can affect your behaviour, relationships, sleeping and eating patterns, and your whole attitude towards living.

Events that can trigger depression include the breakup of a relationship, the death of a loved one and losing a job. Sometimes it has no specific cause, but may occur in older people due to a perceived loss of control in life. The prospect of aging may in itself be a cause of depression, especially in societies that are youth-orientated.

▾ Consider seeking help from a therapist if depression lingers for more than two weeks.

self-help

If you are feeling depressed, ensure that you continue to eat and sleep properly, and that your diet is high in C and B vitamins, essential fatty acids and unrefined carbohydrates. Avoid relying on bad habits such as drinking and drugs – they are false friends.

Exercise regularly – endorphins released during physical activity can help combat depression. Herbalists recommend taking St. John's wort tablets; aromatherapists value rose, neroli, clary sage and bergamot oils.

Don't be afraid to talk to friends and family. Try to explore with them your anxieties, anger and sadness. It is always easier to cope with problems when you can talk about them.

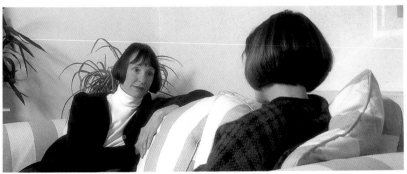

39 re-addressing stress

Stress can chip away stealthily at your health and happiness. Learning how to deal with it successfully will help you towards a lengthy and more satisfying life.

Research has shown that stress can have a profound impact on your health. Stress triggers the "fight or flight" syndrome, in which the body acts as though it is in a life-or-death situation. In this state of physiological arousal, the heartbeat and blood pressure are elevated, and stress hormones such as adrenaline rage through the bloodstream.

If you are constantly under stress, these factors will in time wear down your immune system, making you more susceptible to illness and disease – from common colds to cardio-vascular problems and even cancer.

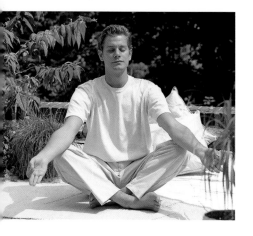

relaxation techniques
Learning relaxation techniques is a powerful antidote to stress. Yoga and meditation help you to centre your thoughts and quiet the mind. Deep breathing helps to oxygenate the cells and relax muscles. Good therapies for releasing tension include massage and aromatherapy. A quick way to beat stress is to go for a walk – exercise uses up adrenaline and brings an endorphin rush that raises the mood, giving a sense of perspective.

re-train your thinking
Trying to think rationally about the causes of stress and anxiety can be helpful. It is often your perception of a situation that makes it stressful, and changing the way you view it can be extremely beneficial.

Make a list of practical things you can do to alleviate a problem, and a list of things that you cannot change. If you have done all that you can, give yourself a break from worry – remind yourself there is no point in fretting.

◀ *Take a deep breath and meditate on the causes of stress and how you can remedy it.*

40 satisfying sex

Important throughout adulthood, sexual activity can be a source of great pleasure, emotional nourishment and spiritual growth. Physical touch brings a confidence that extends to other areas.

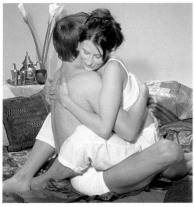

▲ *The intimacy that loving sex brings can provide a solid foundation for happiness.*

Touch is one of the most profound means of communication between two people. The laying of caring hands on the body conveys a depth of feeling that goes way beyond words – it is a direct link to the inner world of feeling, and through it you can express your innermost emotions and desires. People who live with one special partner for a long period – whether married or not – tend to be healthier and live longer. This is partly due to the benefits that regular, loving sex and physical intimacy bring.

increased pleasure

Many people enjoy sex more as they get older, because they have gained experience and confidence. They understand what arouses them and their partner, and are more relaxed about communicating their desires.

The physical changes in sexuality vary. Most people do not notice any major changes until their 50s, when they may experience slower response times. One thing sex researchers agree on is the "use it or lose it" theory – staying sexually active keeps your sex organs functioning and helps maintain sexual desire.

getting closer

To keep long-term relationships alive and meaningful, try exploring different ways to arouse your partner, perhaps using visual stimuli, massage and aromatherapy. Learning about sexual philosophy and technique from different cultures can open deeply fulfilling doors. Tantric sex, from Eastern tradition, takes a holistic view of love and sex where the ultimate aim is for two people to merge spiritually as well as physically.

41 nourishing sleep

Sleep is essential for physical and mental well-being. Although its pattern and quality may change as the body ages, it is an ever-important ingredient for youthfulness and health.

Deep sleep has a tremendous effect on vitality levels. It rejuvenates every cell in the body while resting the nervous system, which in turn is responsible for controlling the digestive, reproductive and immune systems. During sleep, not only are toxins eliminated and tissues rebuilt, but it is believed that the mind works through and helps resolve feelings, problems and challenges through the process of dreaming.

aiding quality sleep

To ensure a deep and restful sleep, the two most important factors are good nutrition and proper exercise. It is best to refrain from caffeine, alcohol and excessive sugar in the evenings – these all exacerbate restlessness and insomnia. Make sure that your bedroom environment is pleasant; that you have a firm bed, fresh air, clean bedclothes and quiet. It can help to take a hot bath an hour before bed; deep breathing and certain yoga poses will also help calm the nervous system.

changing sleep patterns

People may find it more difficult to sleep as they get older, possibly due to the body producing fewer chemicals that control the sleep cycle. Some find that they wake more frequently during the night and spend more time being awake. You can adapt to these natural changes by trying "sleepy" herbal teas before going to bed, or by taking a short nap in the afternoon to augment the sleep cycle.

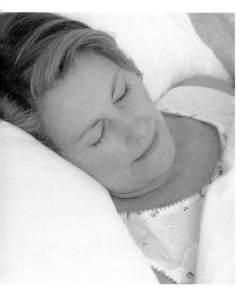

◀ *Sleep patterns change with age – try to discover what schedule works best for you.*

42 healing natural light

Without the sun, there would be no life on Earth – people, plants and animals all move to the rhythm of its rays. Time spent outdoors will keep you in tune with the sun's healing energy.

Sunlight regulates the chemical balance within the pineal gland – without sufficient exposure to the full colour spectrum in sunlight, the finely balanced chemical reactions in the body tend to falter, leaving it prone to ill health. Spending time outside every day will renew your stamina and raise your spirits. Remember always to apply sun cream.

dawn to dusk

Experiments have shown that, as the sun rises, its red light increases pulse, blood pressure and breathing rate, stimulating the body into alertness. These functions are further increased in orange light and reach their peak in yellow light when the sun is high in the sky. Similarly, when the sky turns to subduing blues and greens at dusk, the vital signs decrease and the body prepares for relaxation and sleep.

modern hazard

Many people have jobs that keep them indoors in harsh commercial lighting – this is often produced by white fluorescent tubes, which exclude some of the colours in the

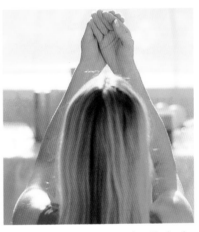

▲ Time spent in the sun energizes the body.

spectrum. If you must work inside, full-spectrum lights are healthier than fluorescent lights – they reduce irritability and promote productivity.

SAD season

The lack of sunlight during the long winter months changes the mood of most people. But for some, Seasonal Affective Disorder (or SAD) causes depression and low energy that only subside at the onset of spring. Women are more prone to SAD because of their complex hormonal makeup.

43 positive thinking

The rumour is true: maintaining a positive outlook not only enhances but prolongs life and increases health. Septuagenarians all agree that looking on the bright side is one of the secrets of new youth.

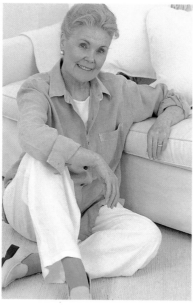

▲ *Look for ways to learn from every situation and you'll find satisfying solutions.*

Some people are more susceptible than others to slipping into negative thinking patterns – perhaps learned unconsciously from family, friends or the media. But by perpetuating a pessimistic outlook – such as always dwelling on what you lack – you may be wasting precious days and years feeling irritated, dissatisfied and unhappy instead of savouring all the wonderful joys of life.

nurture optimism
Fostering a sense of optimism for the present and future has huge benefits for psychological and physical health. Optimism can be enhanced by keeping busy – doing things that make you feel happy and enthused, setting new goals and meeting new people who encourage your positivity.

As we get older, a surplus of negative experiences – bad career moves, failed relationships, illness – may at times threaten to overwhelm us. You can move past these hardships by clearing your mind of emotional baggage from the past – visualize yourself throwing these "bags" away, leaving room for new experiences.

COUNT YOUR BLESSINGS
Begin the day in a positive frame of mind by making a list of five things for which you are grateful. As the days go by, you will see that you have more going for you than you realized.

44 life-affirming spirituality

You needn't be a member of an organized religion to explore your spirituality. Thinking about why you exist and what you are doing is an important part of living a long and meaningful life.

In today's materialistic Western society, it is sometimes easy to forget about the "invisible" life of the soul. When wrapped up in career, family and personal dramas or striving for material gains, you can forget that you are just one piece in a very vast puzzle. Taking time to reflect on your place in the universe can help you lead a more fulfilling life, whether you believe in a god or gods, or simply put your faith in the connections between people.

inner work

Scheduling time every day to think, meditate, pray or just "be" with yourself can help you live more comfortably with the changes that are inevitable for everyone. You may want to consider what happens after death, why events happen in the order that they do, why certain people have come into your life and what you can learn from them. Do you believe in free will or fate, or perhaps a combination of the two?

Knowing where you stand on these complex spiritual issues will help you make informed decisions; even though you may not have all the answers, at least you will be equipped with the tools to try and understand life more fully.

group spirituality

Many people find fulfilment by belonging to an organized faith that dictates a system of set principles and guidelines for living. Exploring the tenets of other faiths may help you to clarify your own views; you may also discover the positive similarities that exist between them all.

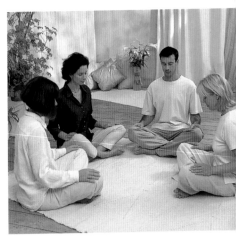

▲ Meditating with others can bring you closer to understanding the meaning of life.

45 creative fun

Having fun is a most underrated activity: from
playfulness and fun have come some of the
world's greatest inventions and works of art –
as well as the most joyous personal pleasure.

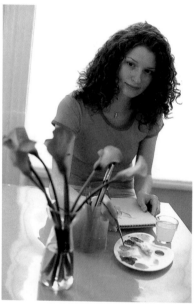

▲ Relax and explore your creative side – the
results might surprise you.

explore strange new worlds

There is so much more to life than
just your current situation – your
home, work environment, city or
village. By exploring different sides
of yourself in a creative activity, you
can expand your whole perspective of
yourself and other people. The sense
of accomplishment that comes from
creating something from nothing
may astound you – it will boost your
confidence in all areas.

If you've always wanted to try
pottery, cooking, saxophone-playing
or creative writing, for example, now
is the time to start. Find a course or
other like-minded people who will
learn to create with you, or get books
and tapes and begin on your own.

don't be shy

Even if you think you won't become
the greatest genius of all time in your
chosen medium, don't let it stop you
from beginning. Creativity is partly
skill, partly unknown quantity – as
any poet will tell you, there is a point
when "something else" takes over and
you're left with a little piece of magic
to take back to the everyday world.

Watch a child play with wooden
blocks or let loose with finger paints –
there's no doubt that having fun is
directly linked with creativity. The
greatest artists are daydreamers, so
allow yourself to gaze into space; you
may be surprised at what you can
accomplish after a break from "reality".

To give yourself a **rejuvenating** new look, experiment with clothes in **styles** and **colours** you wouldn't normally **choose**. Consign items you haven't worn for a **year** to a **charity shop.**

47 uplifting music therapy

There is nothing so moving as music – its effects on the body and soul vary endlessly, from encouraging healing feelings of catharsis to promoting a sense of ageless ecstasy.

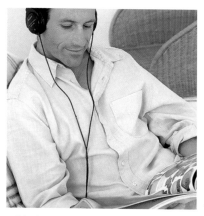

▲ Music can recall people, times and places rather like an emotional history book.

People use music every day as a therapy without even realizing it. When feeling melancholy, depressed or anxious, playing a recording of your favourite music lifts your mood instantly. Music can magnify positive emotions you are feeling as well; taking the journey from the first note of a song to the last is like an enjoyable workout for the psyche.

Playing a musical instrument exercises the brain and co-ordinates thought processes, helping to keep the mind sharp. With the pleasure and satisfaction that performing brings, comes a rush of endorphins, the brain's "feel-good" chemicals.

all together now

Drum circles, choir singing or playing instruments with a group can bring social, emotional and spiritual benefits – as well as increased physical health. Researchers have found that such activities strengthen the immune system; they raise levels of antibodies in the body, helping to fight disease.

Tibetan singing bowls offer music therapy even non-musicians can play. The tuned bowls are played by circling the rims with a mallet; the resulting sound fosters great mental focus.

▼ The sound waves produced by Tibetan singing bowls create healing vibrations.

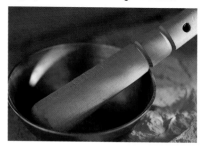

48 strengthening meditation

Anti-aging experts agree that meditation provides a sense of harmony that not only prolongs life, but improves its quality greatly. Here, visualizing a colour is used to balance the mind and emotions.

1 Slowly close your eyes and imagine yourself sitting in a green meadow near a cool, crystal-clear stream, with fragrant flowers surrounding you. The day is clear and bright, with a soft, gentle breeze swirling around you. The sky is blue with soft, white drifting clouds.

2 Choose a colour that you feel helps your sense of well-being. Look at one of the clouds above you, and let this cloud become suffused with your chosen colour. Watch it start to shimmer with its own sparkling light.

3 Allow the cloud to float over you; as it does, it releases a colourful shower of delicate, misty stars that sparkle all around your body and your being.

4 The mist settles on your skin, gently absorbing into your very core, completely saturating your system with its potent healing and strengthening vibrations.

5 Allow the colour to run through your body and your bloodstream for 3–4 minutes, soothing and restoring a sense of well-being. Feel the new pulse of energy in your cells.

6 Allow your pores to open and release the coloured vapour, taking any toxins or draining bad feelings with it. When the vapour runs clear, you can close your pores.

7 Sit quietly with your energized and balanced body for a few moments. Take three deep breaths, releasing each gently, before opening your eyes.

▼ *Regular meditation can bring an oasis of self-contained serenity to a hectic lifestyle.*

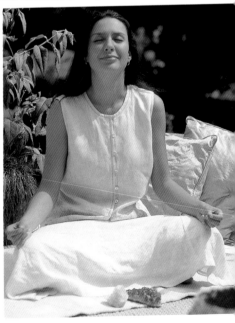

49 go wild

When you feel that life has become monotonous and you are stuck in a loop, trying something new and different will change your perspective, adding youthful excitement and sparkle.

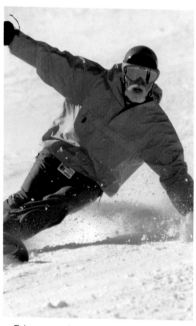

▲ Bring new adventure to your life with a sport such as snowboarding or skiing.

be a daredevil

If you are fit and eager, there is no reason not to try a new sport. Take up ice-skating, bowling, surfing, skiing – or if you enjoy an adrenaline thrill, extreme sports such as skydiving, hang-gliding or white water rafting.

In addition to being challenging and fun, they are a great way to meet new friends. Instruction is advised before beginning any of these activities.

Of course, you don't have to throw yourself down a mountain to go wild, you could sign up for tango lessons, dye your hair a different colour, paint your house pink or throw a large party – the possibilities are endless.

new sensations

Holidays are important, not only as a break from work, but as a refreshing change from normal routine. Visiting new places and cultures puts one's own life in perspective, and home tends to look more appealing on return. You may want to try a package holiday geared towards your interest, whether it's an art break in Paris or an African safari adventure.

If you are dissatisfied in your career, or just always wanted to learn about astrophysics, hairdressing, archeology or art, why not "go back to school"? It is never too late to explore new avenues and broaden your knowledge, for your career, or simply for your own interest.

50 essential relationships

People make the world go round – the longest and happiest lives are filled with friends and loved ones. Always make time for others, and you will share rewards that will delight and nurture your soul.

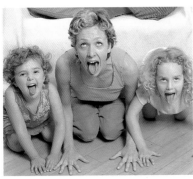

▲ Children understand fun instinctively, and the youngest adults never outgrow it.

different ages

Cultivate friendships with people of different ages and you will never want for new perspectives. Every age group has something to offer – from babies to great-grandads. Older people often bring surprising insights to situations and conversations; younger people have an optimism that is contagious – sharing their sense of hope can make life so much more enjoyable.

family life

Blood ties are among the closest relationships you will ever have, so it is a good idea to make the best of them if you can. Your shared history with a favourite aunt, uncle, brother or sister who has known you since you were three years old can provide a sense of continuity that is unique. Staying close and providing mutual support lends you both a confidence that will help you weather life's storms and heighten its pleasures.

furry friends

Interacting with the animal kingdom – whether in nature or at home – is important for many people. Adopting a pet can add much joy and comfort to your life.

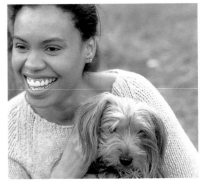

▲ Woman's (and man's) best friend: dogs repay human kindness many times over.

index

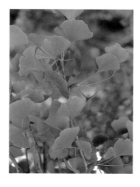
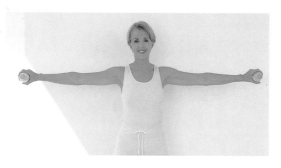

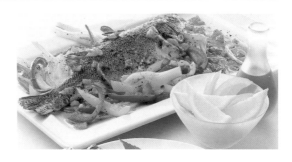

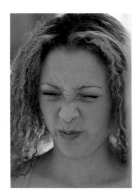

This edition is published by Lorenz Books, an imprint of Anness Publishing Ltd, Hermes House, 88–89 Blackfriars Road, London SE1 8HA; tel. 020 7401 2077; fax 020 7633 9499

www.lorenzbooks.com; www.annesspublishing.com

If you like the images in this book and would like to investigate using them for publishing, promotions or advertising, please visit our website www.practicalpictures.com for more information.

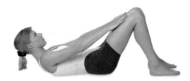

UK agent: The Manning Partnership Ltd; tel. 01225 478444; fax 01225 478440; sales@manning-partnership.co.uk
UK distributor: Grantham Book Services Ltd; tel. 01476 541080; fax 01476 541061; orders@gbs.tbs-ltd.co.uk
North American agent/distributor: National Book Network; tel. 301 459 3366; fax 301 429 5746; www.nbnbooks.com
Australian agent/distributor: Pan Macmillan Australia; tel. 1300 135 113; fax 1300 135 103; customer.service@macmillan.com.au
New Zealand agent/distributor: David Bateman Ltd; tel. (09) 415 7664; fax (09) 415 8892

ETHICAL TRADING POLICY
Because of our ongoing ecological investment programme, you, as our customer, can have the pleasure and reassurance of knowing that a tree is being cultivated on your behalf to naturally replace the materials used to make the book you are holding. For further information about this scheme, go to www.annesspublishing.com/trees

Publisher's note:
The reader should not regard the recommendations, ideas and techniques expressed and described in this book as substitutes for the advice of a qualified medical practitioner or other qualified professional. Any use to which the recommendations, ideas and techniques are put is at the reader's sole discretion and risk.